T0165017

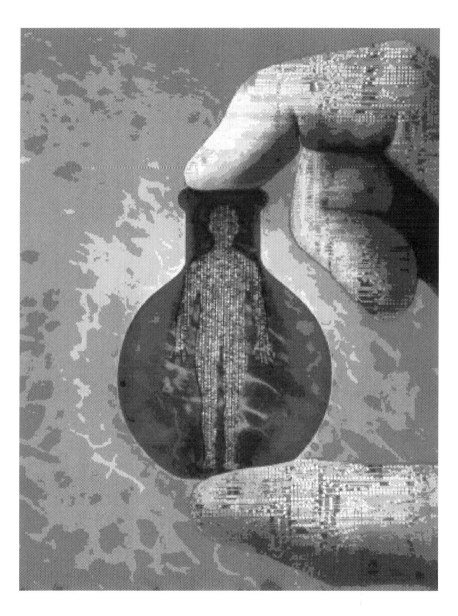

METHODS AND ADVANCES
IN
BIOTECH
Dr. MORTAGY RASHED

Contents

Introduction

Technology is the methods and expertise, knowledge and scientific applications, which bring community needs throughout the ages. We have a tremendous technological development after the industrial revolution the world for the development of new, a new danger is a qualitative shift in the science of electrons minutc, and the evolution occurring in the research and applications of space and, more seriously, what happens in genetic engineering . Relapse dangers of genetic engineering on an equal footing with the benefits being used engineering techniques. Genetic in creating different types of bacteria for the production of hormones such as human insulin, as well as viral proteins for use in the production of vaccines later. We see tremendous progress in the research of gene makes us feel puzzled, every day we discover new, but that the great successes achieved by the science in the field of communicating quickly dropped the line between what we can do today, and we appreciate him for the moment, between the present and Mammal to do tomorrow. Take, for example, procreation find the issues   that worry biological yesterday no longer hold their attention, or perhaps become a priority in their present research , as there is great difference between the means used by the science of birth control and minimize reproduction in the middle of this century, for example, between the sophisticated technology that enables us to control the genetic characteristics of embryos in this day. Eight great achievements in the field of biology and genetic engineering is no longer limited impact on the manufacture of genetically or formation genetic characteristics of human beings, but it has gone for that to include the feelings and self aspects that instinct by .. What you that the issues of pregnancy and childbearing is no longer subject to traditional vaccination, because modern techniques keeping eggs example, transport and planting in the wombs of women Chance had facilitated us many options, we opened the door to alternatives were unthinkable until recently one has been able rights in the near future to create copies thanks to technical uniformity quite sophisticated, allowing it to vaccinate female ovum the somatic cell and not nationality. The fungal and congenital diseases and disabilities, it can eliminate or mitigate the impact of years at least, through controlling gene for the disease as genetic or impairments resulting from the flaw affects the reform of the same gene defect before the birth of the fetus would eliminate those diseases and disabilities—that science unsophisticated and technology are now pose on the scene in recent decades, the problems of moral concern and deserves reflection Devin For as much as to the outcome of our knowledge and increase our ability to control things and allow us new options always IHL also raise new issues revolve around what is right and what is wrong. The criteria identify right and wrong it turned stem from the actual needs of Rights does not necessarily from the traditional sources. In an era of science explosive In this era of advanced technology, has become a touchstone of the complex morality approaching slowly from the reality of the situation that already exists rather than ideals paradox. Indeed, it would not have to change our ethical and turn it not for the era we live variable is already causing significant shift speed. Indeed humanity lived

Recently and still live revolutions in various fields of science impending rights achievements in the fields of corn, electronics, and the conquest of space, but the biology is a scientific revolution in the present day. Through this study on the topic of biotechnology will focus on the two important issues, which raise the interest of scientists and researchers in this age are: 1) genetic engineering (gene). 2) infection.

MORTAGY RASHED

Genetic Engineering

Genetic engineering is a part of the biological revolution in modern evolution passed through four basic stages : 1) Phase biological phones. 2) Phase molecular biology. 3) The stage of genetic engineering. 4) a vital called cloning. The scientists realized the importance of genetics discovery of the nature or inherited gene, to change a lot of appearances and hereditary diseases, in 1953 discovered the nature of this gene at the hands of (James Watson) and (Craig Francis), where it became clear to them that (DNA) molecule consisted of two series complementary of sugar and phosphate and nitrogenous bases, and take these two tapes form snails. There are certain points converge each All the other tape carries full information necessary to control the building of proteins required to guide the vital operations of the total interaction leads in the end to the organism. When the cell divided and separated two series attracts each of the chemical elements of nitrogenous bases is completed, and give us a new structure of peaceful Cyclones double. In this way, the cell maintains the new genetic codes found in the mother cell. It was this discovery significant role in founding the science of genetic engineering and the emergence of the reestablishment of (DNA) or control genes, arriving after the so-called therapeutic vital.

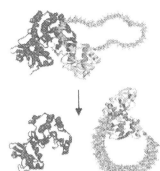

Our group employs molecular biology and genetic engineering techniques for the design and production of proteins by recombinant microbes. Current research include production and purification of CGTase

Researchers:
P.M. Dr. Rosli Md Illias

Laboratory:
Genetic Engineering Laboratory

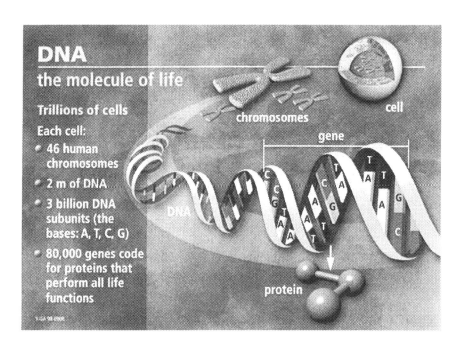

DNA
the molecule of life

Trillions of cells
Each cell:
- 46 human chromosomes
- 2 m of DNA
- 3 billion DNA subunits (the bases: A, T, C, G)
- 80,000 genes code for proteins that perform all life functions

chromosomes

cell

gene

DNA

protein

Gene Technology

Gene technologies, the future of human genetic engineering has made strides and made harvests scientifically unique promise to remove worries and disease, millions of people and opened new horizons in the way of treatment and diagnosis, possibly change the face of the map health early in the next century, especially in the field of diagnosis and treatment of genetic disease and cancer and the diagnosis of viral diseases and genetic testing. A gene therapy (GENE THERAPY) diseases result of the technology revolution gene (GENE TECHNOLOGY) and the accurate knowledge of the installation of genes in the chromosomes (colored objects), which carry genetic characteristics of the human person and include every molecule in his body, whether color of eyes or hair color ,length or various other attributes in addition to the findings of modern science to specific enzyme (RESTRICTION ENZYMES) can be explored genes responsible for the human qualities of each individual and whether to remove pathogens, as well as a gene transfer systems (GENE TRANSFER SYSTEM), which can transport genes to the desired rights. Genes have two : 1) the production of materials for the continuation of the life of cells. 2) production of materials needed body such as insulin and various hormones and correct the error, which happens to these genes lead to the correct track, and therefore the possibility of cure hereditary diseases, it is clear that gene therapy in its simplest form is to introduce genes and functional (FUNCTIONAL GENE) to the cells of the patient to replace the genes infected either because of a genetic disease or unearned. Through DNA analysis, which holds rights within the body can map gene everyone has been identified about 40 thousand genes hereditary while the goal is access to knowledge between 75-100 A. genes, through the huge project funded by the United States and cost three billion dollars and employ hundred plant and will be attended by several countries in the world. The gene map is a way designed to identify qualities rights and good vision allowing know the true picture and full respect for all human health in terms of growth and development, diagnosis and subsequent treatment future in the light of genetics and the discovery of individuals who are willing to certain diseases and work in every way to prevent morbidity and preventive methods on the environment in some cases because the disease is not as a result of genetic factors, but the result of the interaction of genetic factors and environment as exposure to radiation, pesticides and some medicines, cigarette smoke and other factors motivating. The past years have witnessed dozens of attempts to cure gene For example : During the 1994 (the inauguration) is the first real beginning and promising to develop what was known with a suicide gene therapy for cancer, and scientists expect that the great revolution happening in the future in dealing with cancer, after they achieved very good results at the level of principle with certain types skin cancer, as Ironically, scientists are strong indications that the possibility of success with cancer of the gastrointestinal tract, throat and esophagus tumors and diseases of the contract deployed sporadically in the human body. In a nutshell, the idea of gene therapy to introduce similar time bomb in tumor cells where explode once Docking cancer cell lead to the crash of cancerous cells or genes to cancer cells make toxic materials sorted and thus the crash itself …

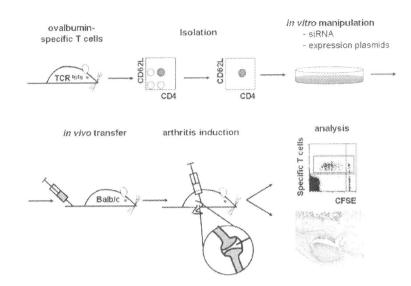

ovalbumin-specific T cells

Isolation

in vitro manipulation
- siRNA
- expression plasmids

in vivo transfer

arthritis induction

analysis

Experimental system for the functional gene analysis in T cells in in vivo disease models. T cells derived from TCR-tg/tg mice can be transfected in vitro to overexpress or knockdown a previously identified target gene. The modified T cells populations can be transferred into non-transgenic cells and the effect of the gene modification on the antigen-specific immune reaction and disease development can directly be analysed.

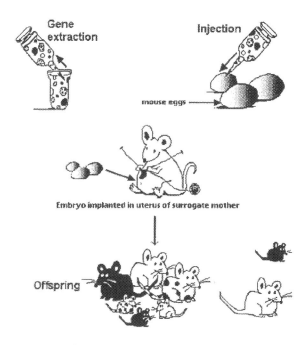

Transgenic Mice

Illustration of how transgenic mice are produced.

Genes responsible for particular traits or disease susceptibility are chosen and extracted. Next they are injected into fertilized mouse eggs. Embryos are implanted in the uterus of a surrogate mother. The selected genes will be expressed by some of the offspring.

Since the first gene transfers into mice were successfully executed in 1980, transgenic mice have allowed researchers to observe experimentally what happens to an entire organism during the progression of a disease. Transgenic mice have become models for studying human diseases and their treatments.

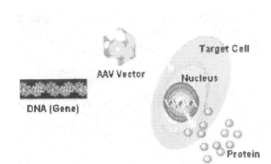

Sure enough, the treatment produced lasting improvement in the animals. After the gene therapy, blood-clotting times dropped from more than an hour's time to 15 to 20 minutes. Normal clotting time in healthy animals is about six minutes. It took about two months for the genes to maximize expression of the missing protein. The researchers were encouraged to find that expression levels remained stable for more than a year after the one-time treatment. Moreover, no side effects or limiting immune responses occurred as a result of treatment.

Prostate Cancer

Prostate cancer : the method for the treatment of prostate cancer surgery ,radiotherapy or hormonal.Surgical treatment is the extermination of the prostate island or radiotherapy is the best way deep in the early stages of treatment, in the case of the spread of the disease to parts of the body in the form of both high schools in thc system or lymph glands or other body parts are treatment the use of hormones, and using this method will control the disease for a long time, but if there colonies of cancer cells are not sensitive to Hormones, leading to the spread of the disease again. The pace of genetic therapy is a big step in the direction of overcoming carcinomas which afflict many prostate. Where, a team of scientists to find a new vaccine was prepared in the methods of genetic engineering are expected to have an effective influence in helping patients with this type of cancer who have not responded to conventional treatment methods. This method relies on the amendment recipes cancerous cells from secondary tumors by infusing new vaccine to turn cancerous cells from the elements urges object to the composition of objects existing anti-cancer by leading to the break the growth of secondary cancers and places its inception in prostate During testing researchers have found a gene activated responses immune system has been encouraged cells to kill cancer cells and then planted inside the skin of rats suffering from prostate cancer and later became mice able to get rid of the cancerous cells and when they are approved this treatment system on humans, it will save millions of patients who suffer or died of prostate cancer every year.

Detection of Cancer Cells Directly

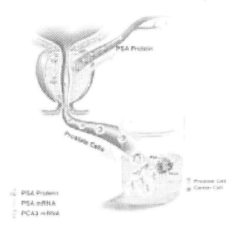

Diagram showing urinary PCA3 (lower arrow) vs serum PSA (upper arrow) Whereas PSA is a glycoprotein that may enter the bloodstream, PCA3 is a gene that exists in the nuclear material of prostate epithelial cells which may be shed into the urine. Those cells, if cancerous, over-express the gene. That over-expression, which may be many times that found in benign prostate cells, is detected by the assay. Importantly, PCA3 expression is normalized against a background of prostate specific nuclear material (PSAmRNA), yielding a PCA3 score The PCA3 score is much more cancer-specific than serum PSA levels which are confounded by factors such as prostate volume, age, trauma, and certain drugs.

Tay-Sachs

Tay-Sachs : introduced genetic engineering technique in the prevention of genetic diseases to the beginning of the 1990s .. In 1989 an American woman gave birth to a child suffers from a rare disease and very strange known as (Tay-Sachs) affects members of the body and the brain as a result of a congenital defect inherited leads to the symptoms of severe and devastating ended in the death of the child and through examination of the father and mother found they sphere for gene causes the disease and thus the likelihood of injury to children arriving the same disease list.. resorted to a doctor in 1993 to test for genes can be made of the sperm that have been vaccinated ectopic father and mother through this test and sperm in the first test phase consisting of eight cells can be examined through gene know whether the child next suffering from the disease are disposed of sperm prior to their encampment, in the womb or sound completely fed sperm in the uterus for pregnancy and supplements the child is born naturally.. and the parents have agreed to conduct the experiment and examine the genes in the sperm cells of the eight have already been fertilized in vitro were taken from mother by spermatozoa father outside the uterus as is done in the case of a child pipes and when sperm were divided into eight cells were genetic testing shows that three of the embryos are completely free of disease genes (Tay) has been planting them and it was placed into the womb to grow and bigger, and nine months later was the birth of a healthy child for start a new page in the history of medicine is a change in the format and method of treatment for inherited diseases.

Brain with Tay-Sachs Disease

Hexosaminidase deficiency with accumulation of clear to foamy ganglioside neurons.

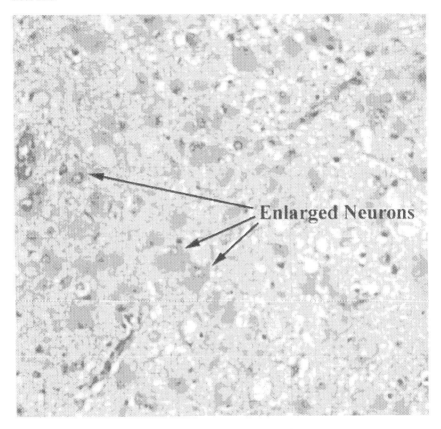

Enlarged Neurons

Genetic testing

Genetic testing: The genetic tests of the fastest growth areas in the science of medical diagnosis, thanks to the achievements of the draft HUMAN GENOM PROJECT have been identified, installation and isolate many of the genes responsible for hereditary diseases such as CYSTIC FIBROSIS anemia and HUNTINGTON CHOREA genetic commonly suffer from about 500 thousand people in the United States alone .. and who are asymptomatic at age forty or more through the emergence of bags and Vesicles in the kidneys, liver, pancreas and spleen and lead to inflation and possibly total renal failure involves genetic tests on a wide range of methods used to search for the existence of genes in cells or measurement .. and the effectiveness of these methods depends on the number of chromosomes in the cells of the patient or measuring the quantity of proteins in the blood of the patient Scouts or analyze genetic material of cells by molecular pathways can detect the genetic sequence qualitative one between three million pairs rules which form human genome material Currently there are four types of tests genetic : 1)AMINOCENTESIS : personal being tested after 10 weeks of pregnancy as taking some cells from the fluid tubercular order an examination to test the biological abnormality in the chromosomes . 2) CHORIONIC VILLUS SAMPLING: testing principles after 10 weeks of pregnancy, where some cells take developing placenta countries to examine chromosomes. 3) COELOCENTESIS: talk test-not yet adopted-being before 10 weeks of pregnancy. Where some cells taken from the cavity that surrounds the Earth and tubercular to examine chromosomes. 4) PREIMPLANTATION: test installation of genetic material (DNA) of the embryos at the stage of the eight cells to detect the presence of certain genetic defects. It allowed not genetic testing to preschool birth but can be used to diagnose genetic deformities in either children or adults. Applying these genetic tests can predict the course of the patient's health and warn of the danger of being sick .. And if it was a combination of genetic tests hoped that the treatment the defective gene and gene functional sound, it will be able to these tests lead to a real cure.

Distinguishing features of the PCA3 assay (Gen-Probe, Inc.) are shown in sequence.

In **step No.1** (top), target capture of the mRNA is performed, using magnetic bead (purple).

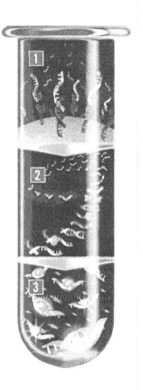

In **step No. 2**, the captured gene is amplified using Transcription-Mediated Amplification, a process that generates some 10 billion copies of PCA3 in one hour.

In **step No. 3**, the Hybridization Protection Assay is performed using DNA probes tagged with a chemiluminescent substance that is activated upon contact with detection reagents.Details of the assay are described in a recent publication10.

Gene Treatment

Gene treatment for obesity : Some might imagine that the matter was exaggerated to a large degree Could large and serious diseases such as AIDS, cancer, heart disease, Ebola and other diseases and epidemics of new and old that have returned to plague the world and viciousness and brutality to cast their dark shadow on the future rights to interested people and the world's media discovered the (gene), which cause human obesity. The effects of the news published in the journal (Nature) Scientific American a huge fuss, in the United States, Britain, Russia and the rest of the Western world, it was announced Researchers Institute (Howardhead) Medical University of New York (Rockefeller) they managed to isolate the gene that causes obesity in mice, as well as they had found a similar gene in the fatty tissues of humans, which holds promise for an imminent treatment crucial to the problem of overweight and get rid of excess fat. The idea of discovery, in a nutshell, that Dr. (Jeffrey Friedman), a group of researchers with the Institute had been able to reduce the weight of several mice fat (by 30%) by infusing new hormone that controls body weight. In addition to reducing the weight of the number of mice fathead then rates have declined cholesterol and Glucose, which had hit a low of diabetes. In spite of the uproar that followed the dramatic discovery, it is still early to put every confidence that hormone with that laboratory tests proved successful. Had everything proceeded on track, it was offensive into practical use by five to ten years until a body of American food and medicine to be used after to make sure that the hormone not cause man harmful side-effects.. In sum, the future of gene medicine, reports in May 1994 indicating that the gene therapy technique depends primarily to replace gene replace another in the hope that it is supplying the body with a therapeutic impact. 1) Gene sound of the cell is charged to the private vehicle (one of viruses) as a transition. 2) One of the vehicles is to enter the cell nucleus ailing. 3) The new gene, which injects itself into the cell where the patient begins his work in protein production required. 4) Through cell cultivation of the new gene will be produced billions of copies that are injected in the patient there will be a cure.

Among the targets for the future treatment of genetic diseases following :-1) Hemophilia :-a disease that affects only men and the resulting imbalance in the genetic characteristics causing liquidity and infected blood disease hemophilia patients can be treated by intravenous formulations containing coagulation factors help at the first signs of Bloodying (hemorrhage), but doses of containing Group genotype (gene) causes Coagulation is the easiest way to control the disease.2) Diabetes :-stems from the inability of the pancreas to produce sufficient quantities of the hormone insulin regulating Glucose levels in the blood is a genetic disease begin to appear when the death of cells that produce this hormone, located within the pancreas and the new method of treatment requires patients to give one of the enzyme (GMD), so accustomed to the body's immunity the existence of these enzymes and coexistence with them. Previously, a number of tests on rats infected diabetic The result was stopped on the body building objects countermeasures to resist these enzymes proved after (40) weeks that rats freed from diabetes and had exposed him once again. 3) Diseases of aging:-Recent research demonstrated that the symptoms of aging occur as a result of the lack of natural secretions tomorrow Adrenal after age (25) years and had been isolated molecule, which makes these secretions, which allows a pharmaceutical production. It is scheduled to begin soon on the experience of this medication (100) of the elderly volunteers, At the same time, other research will be to determine the possible relationship between this molecule and each of cancer and AIDS. 4) Parkinson's disease:-an advanced state of central nervous system disorders and it happens because the gradual disintegration of brain cells that produce a vital chemical known as (dopamine), but injected doses of cell-producing altered intravenous unsuccessful, but scientists devise method is successful in this regard.

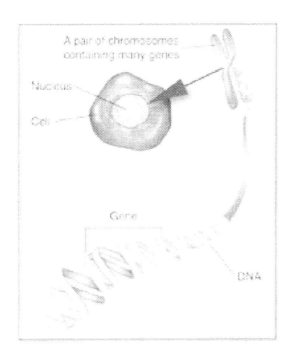

A pair of chromosomes
containing many genes

Nucleus

Cell

Gene

DNA

Genes affect a person's risk of developing diabetes.

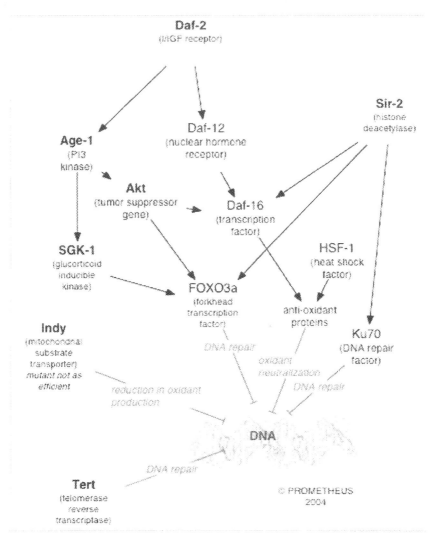

LONGEVITY GENES AND DNA REPAIR

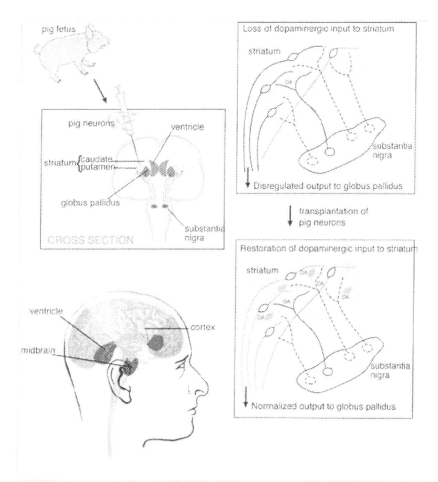

Treatment of Parkinson's disease by transplantation of pig neurons. *a*, Cells are obtained from the mesencephalic brain region of fetal pigs under optimized conditions for cell survival. This region contains dopaminergic neurons, as well as other neural and glial cells. A total of 1.2×10^7 cells in 240 µl (from 15-20 pig fetuses) is injected into the striatum on one side of the Parkinson patient's brain, with the patient conscious and using local anesthesia. *b*, Parkinson patients suffer from a loss of dopaminergic neurons in the substantia nigra, which sends processes into the striatum. This results in insufficient release of dopamine (DA) in the striatum onto neurons projecting to the globus pallidus or the substantia nigra. The result is loss of movement control, rigidity and tremor. *c*, Transplantation of pig neurons into the striatum potentially restores dopaminergic synaptic inputs onto neurons projecting out of the striatum and allows resumption of normal movements.

Genetic Engineering And Environment

Genetic engineering and the environment :-every day new developments emerge and impressive achievements in the field of technology, an area vital research .. I mean trying to improve the capabilities of living organisms through pooling characteristics of many types are often very different. The game moving genes from one organism to be separated and injected in the cell of another organism. To become cell more new capacity to produce different vehicles or carrying out controversial surprisingly have never exercised over the years. This is exactly the essence of genetic engineering and sinew .. Synthetic materials for plastics, for example Ka has become an important part in our lives is hard to ignore, since it was well... Recent research has paid attention to try to produce new vehicles similar in denaturalization vehicles Plastic However, it difficult the microbial digestion... So that the closure of one life cycles. Indeed, the researchers find in a chemical empire in England to discover one super strains layers ability to convert sugar to (polyester) in the semi-bacterial qualities natural plastic material to a large extent. The scientists used genetic engineering this miracle microbe and went on to develop through the transfer of new genetic mechanism to ensure production and abundant (polyester) promised to replace the plastic. The really surprising that ecologists have expressed their welcome new microbe, it is a digestible bacterial, mere samples of it buried in the soil, to break away completely after a period similar to the period required to analyze the paper. We have sent a science of genetic engineering scientists hope to the environment in the production of alternative materials for synthetic materials, but materials are natural microbial digestion and entry into the natural life cycle without pollution.

While microbes ferment organic material into polymer form naturally, Metabolic has introduced metabolic engineering that enables technicians to create microbes with better fermentation characteristics, or a better microbial "biofactory." Existing microbes can be tuned to give better product yield and produce useful polymers from inexpensive feeds.

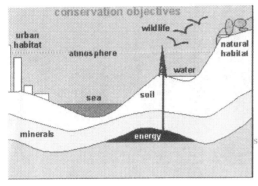

Nevertheless, it seems that the three underlying causes, **population growth**, **economic growth** and **material needs** ('standard of living') are too holy to be stemmed, or even discussed. So it happens that all our conservation efforts are directed at fixing problems, rather than preventing them. Worse still, the concept of **sustainable development** requires us to increase economic activity while also conserving the environment, two opposing goals. Conservationists now try to improve our 'quality of life', the need for a clean environment, such as clean air and water, uncluttered living areas, and unspoiled scenic lands. Only very recently has the concept of **biodiversity** entered the conservationist's vocabulary. It requires healthy ecosystems, not just for the benefit of people but also for those other millions of species. Conservation can be grouped into the following classes:

Problem solving:

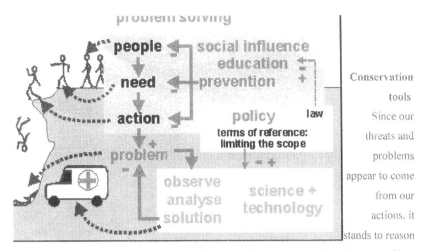

that controlling those, would bring solution. However, the path to a problem consists of several steps, which can all be addressed to solve or to alleviate our problems. The diagram here shows that problems arise from a need, which leads to action. To look at problems alone, would bring costly fixes that do not last. They look like providing ambulances at the bottom of the cliff, rather than a fence at the top. The best solution is decreasing human population, then abating our needs, followed by controlling our actions, and finally by fixing problems.

Genetic Engineering And Pollution

Genetic engineering and pollution problem : The global stock of freshwater cause for concern really Thus, killing cries scientists demanding everyone's mind and conscience to preserve the precious drop of water. but advocacy of the need to use water again and again through the life cycles of scientists has begun micro-organisms (microbiological) in Educational bacterial strains strange mood where not only grow in sewage .. Thus been reared in tanks inside those huge stores of water and then the bacteria feed on various solid waste and liquid However, these natural bacteria often those who rebel bad life in the sewage we see it strike on the analysis of all the waste and complete analysis then we can re-use water treatment only for the purpose of irrigation and agriculture.. Scientists therefore decided to genetic engineering to intervene with these organisms so willingly embrace of several genes and genetic new genotype within its video to make it more capable of swallowing all kinds of waste and more quickly .. but that the material smells opens appetite, and thereby re scientists game biotechnology those new hope in the possibility of restoring water corrections life cycle closed. The Second World War was to come to an end even worked around the globe legend DDT to enter the world in the global war against many insect pests, insects and disadvantages of DDT began unfolding day after day in view of the firmness and strong chemical solubility meager start accumulate in soil and water and slowly emerged adverse impacts on the various neighborhoods bringing one of the symbols of the failure of modern technology in harmony and harmony with nature circular logic—that this dilemma and found a surprising drop us coefficient of genetic engineering .. has been able team of researchers from the reprogramming of some strains of soil bacteria to introduce genes can produce the composite structure of a protein where permitted spatial molecule containing DDT inside cover and isolated from the environment to prevent influence-threatening environment.

Nitrogen Fertilizer

Nitrogen fertilizer :—that there are millions of microorganisms in the soil capable of correcting the imbalance in the balance of nitrogen-the need for inorganic fertilizers. However, the usual rights hopes to reap more food So feed more fertilizer plants, which in turn changed to some absorb nitrate plant to apply in his veins and the other part water leakage and every evil. What leakage of water has become a threat to fish but lost its validity for drinking water when the concentration of nitrates there. Let us image then and now what happens to humans when applied nitrate in the digestive system. There germs normal colon bacteria called disappoint deal with the transformation of nitrate to nitrite, which absorbs compound in the blood to interact with the hemoglobin levels prevent ability to transport oxygen, causing serious illness so-called (Methomogelopenemia), which causes the death of infants and natural disaster occur when vehicles nitrate soil under the influence of anaerobic bacteria since its conversion to Nitro and then to nitrogen oxides carbonated escalate into layers of the atmosphere, where the ozone layer, there is a slow erosion of this class of threats the entire life of that has scientists looking for a solution to restore the ecological balance was logical that these scientists is to develop new plant varieties have the ability to absorb nitrogen from the air directly or through bacterial strains repeat synthesis live with a living symbiotic which inevitably shatter for dispensing with fertilizer industrial, which represents a threat to the environment.

Oil Pollution

Oil pollution :—The environmental scientists in the world knew well CAUTION oil pollution, particularly maritime routes followed by oil tankers be concentrated along the continental shelf in waters off the coast, these are all areas of particular importance to the productivity of the sea, both staple food for marine organisms or products of various economic basic, as these areas are fisheries and traded with high importance, which represents a threat economically and environmentally inevitably now : what can scientists genetic engineering to eliminate the pollution of the sea oil? The truth is that there are many amazing ideas, and one of these ideas adopted by the American company General Electric, when enable researchers to create bacteria capable of engulfing the oil spilled in the waters of the seas and oceans have chosen scientists company three elements of the natural bacteria each with the capacity to devour any partial oil every part or one of the structure. Since the breeding grounds desired to develop bacteria capable of swallowing oil partly, but not a whole has spent in the work crossbreeding kinds of bacteria three minutes painstaking work requiring vaccination of some or transplantation characteristics others and manipulates different genes. and those actions resulted in a new bacterium does not exist in nature, and can swallow whole oil .. The product active for some treatments for biotechnological problems of environmental pollution, both what has been accomplished buildings, which is expected to be completed during the next few years, hints clearly the success in some of these catch the treatments where the laws of nature did not overpowering clash, such treatments were forced to fractures and ruptures one of the flaws in the environmental life while so far failed treatments biotechnology which again find their way to closing sessions of the same environmental efficiency. Thus, the new environmental problems that might result in some of those new treatments than requires necessarily further reflection on the full and continued environmental audit, in the hope of achieving the principle of harmony and harmony with the logic of natural ecological cycles .. and anticipated results will depend on the extent of our understanding of the nature of environmental laws and respect, and that it is an integral whole that indivisible .. and then being placed in this context, the need to test seriously each new step in the field of genetic engineering and testing of the interaction between each organism derived and environmental conditions in the labs before they enter natural environment.

Gene and Food

Gene and food : God created the earth in the balance calculated and furnished in natural resources necessary for life and has given biodiversity, which is the foundation for environmental safety and food security source and economic future generations is lifeline on Earth, but human sought during the past centuries to the welfare and prosperity at the expense of nature and balances breach draining its resources and reports indicate the Food and Agriculture Organization of the United Nations that 25% of all plant and animal species on this planet is threatened by extinction over the next thirty years, which will increase fears about food supplies for future generations. The plant genetic resources is crucial to food security especially since there are products of plant origin estimated at about 13% of the food material benefit of Rights has decided Food and Agriculture Organization said that since the beginning of this century, 75% of the genetic diversity of agriculture crops lost. About 30% of the earth's surface that is free of the ice cover of forests and forest when exposed to the erosion simply removed the numbers more trees are also lost. Reports also indicate the Food and Agriculture Organization indicate that the rate of extinction of animals factions has increased dramatically, and the reason in most cases is higher specialization in the production process of modern livestock. Perhaps Stock genetic erosion in general throughout the world are essentially economic reasons, social and political Consumption of genetic resources are increasingly part of a small and wealthy people in the world in terms of the devastating effects caused by poor people and its desperate struggle for survival on the other hand were two key to destroy the natural genetic sources. and genetic engineering has been characterized in that man for the first time in history has possessed the means to leverage underlying genetic stock in all organisms, whether plant, animal or micro-organisms including satisfy the ambitions of any crew that genetic or genotypes of the images of life can be different that placed on the table of genetic processes to be adapted to surgery for the development of genetic variations in genes known and is a natural result of the evolution of life. As a result of environmental pollution, water shortages and lack of food and desertification all worries of world today. Therefore returned scientists searching for God in the riches of the Earth and genetic sources in the form of plants, animals and microorganisms capable of solving the problems and worries of human and preserves in specialized institutions always stopped in the so-called Bank of genotype or gene bank.

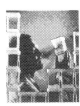

Modern food biotechnology is a refined version of this same process. Today, scientists obtain desired traits by adding or removing plant genes. (Genes are the hereditary units that form the "blueprint" of all living beings. They determine characteristics such as the number of peas in a pod, the color of the flowers, and so on.) For example, scientists can remove a gene for a trait such as dark kernels from one plant and add it to another plant's genetic makeup

Gene Bank

Gene bank : the genetic sources of this and similar bank deposits and balances of the commercial banks. It comprises four main sections bank namely:-1) the exploration and collection of genetic resources, this section based planning and implementation of exploratory missions to locate a genetic source then collected is also receiving genetic sources of genetic other banks. 2) Processing Section textures and crews genetic The Section processing genotypes through isolate genetic material DNA or gene undesirable or chromosomal gene carriers can also be processed in other ways genotypes differ by source type genotype For example in the case of plant genetic resources can be saved or group of cells plant tissue that can evolve under conditions that are suitable for growth to give new plants, seeds or other plant parts as part of the leg, suggested some plant cells, in the case of nitrogen and microbial genetic resources can be conserved in private farms containing glycerol means nitrogen. 3) Section multiplication and evaluation:-and has a crew of genetic propagation and follow-up. 4) The documentation section:-registering and maintaining information on bank balances of genetic sources through the use of computers to facilitate information with other gene banks and facilitate the utilization of genetic resources in collaboration with institutions and scientific institutes specialized. The genotypes and crews distinct genetic cornerstone programs in genetic engineering and genetic sources contained in plant, animal and microbial.

Gene banks store genetic material from plants or animals such as seeds,spores or eggs frozen in cold chambers at minus 20 degrees Celsius, keeping it intact for over 100 years for later use.

Gene Bank

Microbes for The Manufacture of Food

Microbes for the manufacture of food :—There are numerous ways to manipulate genes and gene transfer between organisms is one of the ways we call the technique of DNA(RECOMBINANT DNA) synthesis technique which requires us some reflection and much patience in the test tube filled a few cells to be transferred one of their genes to bacteria and genetic Let us suppose that this gene is gene rennin enzyme production is the same enzyme produced by the cells of the fourth stomach of young calves and used in the manufacture of cheese and then isolating the tape genetic DNA of cells of the stomach fourth Calves are then cut into parts (tape genotype) by special types of enzymes fiery pieces and then confuse this with what can be considered (cart transfer), which in this case small parts of the DNA-called PLASMID In a few enzyme origin (adhesive), which are linked together to produce the hybridization of DNA are then penetration of this hybrid cells in the host bacteria such as E.coli and distribution cells in the laboratory applied and then left to proliferate and become each plant for the production of DNA hostile compiled, which contains a gene production cholinesterase resonance for the first time in history, and all that follows is easy and accessible and known to all the workers in the field of industries fermented Those who combined microbe rate adequate food here and begin the process microbe, it gets copies itself so digest food, and the required output of the new article, which microbe was not known before. The products of this revolution no longer When we look at the value before the market annually from vitamins will not realize the goal of vitamins care when scientists first biotechnological have counted that these products increase in the value of 670 million pounds sterling annually. Thus we genetic engineering scientists engaged in the production of many vitamins from modified micro-organisms, including B12, B2, E, D, and others. Other scientists seek to improve the baking industry by producing microbial strains and more plants with a high level of fermentation and other vehicles another possible production technology such as the ASPARTAM one of the important vehicles in the food industry, like the rule, which could

MONELLIN gene engineering sector in some bacterial strains to reach production more economically. Either the BROMELIN often used by manufacturers to soften meat, scientists succeeded on a commercial scale production of bacteria and genetically address There is a long list of important organic acids such as acetic acid and lactic acid, benzoic acid and other objectives of the revolution are genetic scientists also identified the importance of the production of color and natural dyes such as carotenes by microorganisms repeat genetic synthesis. Thus, we believe we have tried to predict the basic parameters for the future food production and processing those basic parameters on which the chart features these scientists behind the doors laboratories, however imaginary picture of the future world food will remain secret so that genetic engineering is still evolving in the shadows.

Cloning Vital

Cloning vital :-meaning copies or therapeutic cloning is a replica of a living organism, until late 1992 was vital cloning technology CLONING limited to a plant using farms cell and tissue plant and animal world of using replacement organs and genetic technology Copies embryos far removed from the human world, but in late 1993 month advanced world scientific-technological revolution and a new "versions of human embryos" where enable scientists American Secretaries "Jerry Hall" and "Estellman" to reaching a reproduction of the human ovum eggs animals human sperm. But what is the scientific basis for cloning? Can be applied to serious rights? The Ewe cloning "Dolly" the first mammal to be reproduced in order to produce a photograph replica of another animal relying on the deep tissues of this animal and technology, which helped to reproduce that might be used more easily to modify the genetic characteristics of animals and more than that the birth of the "Dolly" questions to answer most of the scientists looking for answers about the role of DNA in the process of growth creatures to become members very full growth and in spite of public concern felt by the scientific and religious media because of the cloned "Dolly" the matter is not new to mankind since tens of years, scientists trying unsuccessfully cloning animals from tissues of individuals of them, as it is known mammal species reproduce in a sexual reproduction and can produce identical copies of a normal except in the case of identical twins, etc. In contrast to many other organisms, mammals amounting can not copy by themselves. The best way to manufacture identical copy of mammal is to reiterate what happens during the process of formation of identical twins in the early stages of growth when the egg divided into a limited number of cells have all identical At the same time, none of them have started after playing any special task growth in the egg at this stage when we separated each cell on each other to be able to grow up to become full members, usually the rights to the twins grow that way naturally unintentional As for the animals, the scientists are deliberately dividing the embryo in the first stages of growth As for the "Dolly" the matter is somewhat different Until now be reproducing mammals through the process of transferring the nucleus. This includes the integration of two cells together: a cell from an individual donor shoulder all characteristics of the DNA during cell ovum is removed DNA from the egg... Is a meticulous process but not difficult and they are frequently over the past years. Once integration the two cells (a process which is usually conducted using electric shocks simple), the resulting cell is transferred to the uterus tenant (SURROGATE) So far, Animal production is subject to growth and life has been possible only through a cell taken from an embryo in the first stages of growth .. The attempts to mammal cloning of cells more mature animals were doomed to failure with genetic defects and chromosomal clear in gene dreams.

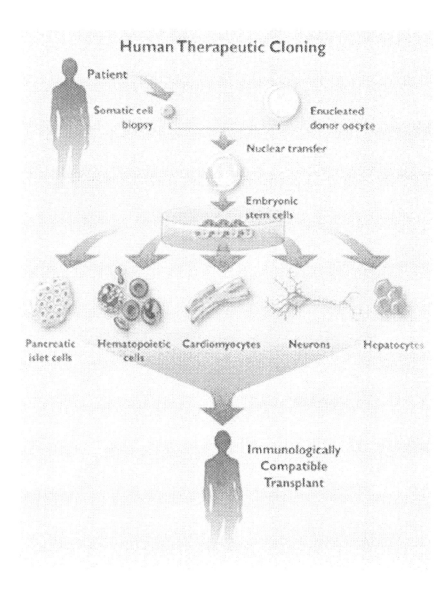

Human Therapeutic Cloning

Patient

Somatic cell biopsy

Enucleated donor oocyte

Nuclear transfer

Embryonic stem cells

Pancreatic islet cells

Hematopoietic cells

Cardiomyocytes

Neurons

Hepatocytes

Immunologically Compatible Transplant

Advanced Cell Technology, Inc., Worcester, Massachusetts.

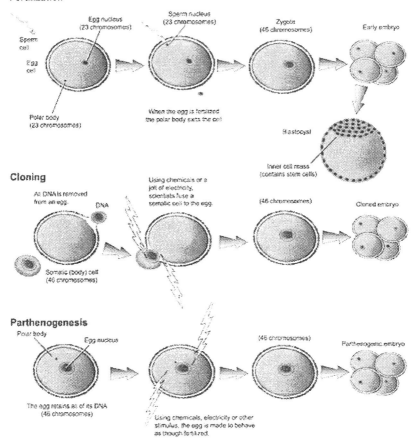

Diagram of early stages of human fertilization, cloning, and parthenogenesis.
[Modified from Rick Weiss and Patterson Clark, *The Washington Post*.]

I t is strange to see many "Dolly" scientific dangerous precedent while it is in fact not the first organism to be created using genetic engineering, and become a modern world and the story of this creation are no more stories raise Domestic lessons gene Transgenic DNA, which has been modified to include their own genes in other animals or to remove genes already become one of the components Established in research labs and biotech companies, this type of animals is considered a test tube alive to allow scientists to establish models diseases rights of the easiest to deal with and try to experiment and to create treatments have larger quantities of proteins useful at lower cost and whether the goats capacity to produce objects mankind can counter the pigs production of materials to help thrombolysis, mice experiments have been carried out to near the medicines of their own DNA from the DNA of humans but for Dolly They enjoyed great fame because of its non-traditional Twenty years ago, almost the first mice were produced by Jenny subsequently became a favorite among researchers injected in the nucleus of human ovum female modern fertilization was carried out those delicate process under the microscope and using needles glass in the accuracy of the greatest injection of DNA with the use of the least possible pressure to stabilize the egg in place until the injection, the scientists hoped to succeed in mice, which are produced in such a way as to the new mice born when they become extremely successful and make this experience there are now about several thousand types of mice produced in this way (lessons gene) to be used in different research purposes. After:-the human genetic engineering has two sides, like every other science, one positive and one negative but the positive side we have been exposed to in this chapter is the goals and objectives sought by the Commissioner of this science to rid mankind of genetic pathologies by changing the genetic code found in embryos and reach types diagnosis The treatment of various cancers and other diseases. The downside is the applications that scientists dreamed of changes of human nature through genetic tampering formulators view access to the so-called giant of man or Superman.

Immunology and AIDS

Immunology and AIDS :-born immunology in the lap of Microbiology and germs While there is a difference of opinion about the starting point of this flag, however, the opinion of many condemns birth to the unique experiences by rural doctors from (Ghlouester Chier) in England and raised for the first time the concept of the body in response to the factors exotic invading object Despite these relatively early birth, the science of immunology independent not only emerge in the 1950s and 1960s when technological development has enabled the identification of anatomical and functional structures of the immune system and show the uniqueness of lymph tissue function commander and coordinator of the immune defense operations. Seldom have the disease in the 20th century was for immune deficiency syndrome AIDS impact on the scientific community and the amazing successes in the eradication of infectious diseases where no longer pose a threat to life and new scientists began converting some effort cancers and diseases that are the result of scientific progress, and this increased the average Construction in developed societies. The result of AIDS knows detailed (acquired Immune Deficiency Syndrome) from obstructed labor human immunodeficiency virus HIV in the central cells of the immune system and destroy these cells called T4 assistance or CD4, which are like the orchestra leader for the Immune coordinate and harmonize between the different immune responses leading to the erosion of the census, these cells gradually to Landing immunological function of the patient is ultimately phase Immune Deficiency respiratory and becomes susceptible to various infections, tumors and has provided innovative techniques scientists accurately on the life cycle of HIV testing is conducted on patients infected with the possible use of antiretroviral drugs for HIV estimate half-life of the virus and the rapid propagation and compensation were found to be HIV take occasional invasion of the cell while generating new viral particles to invade other cells about 2.6 day also estimated the number of viral particles generated daily in these patients by about ten billion viral molecule any rate multiplication of the virus and destroy cells and the high-end over a long period, but what does that mean? How can these facts be a source of optimism? In fact, it further if the defense forces capable of achieving balance with the virus and keep it under control for a period of more than ten years, despite the use of the virus through all this period has spent the reproduction and development, we can upset the balance in favor of final a strong immune and one of two ways : strengthening defenses the body and makes it more ability to produce effective responses to the HIV virus is weakening or make it more vulnerable to these forces, or a combination of both cross Maybe we had to change the mentality that we were dealing with this factor in contravention of the nurse now we have become accustomed during our dealings with other infectious diseases. The researchers will soon have achieved many important discoveries that could have a significant impact on future strategies, especially in the area of prevention and treatment has finally been disclosed, "Assistant acceptant" to secure the entry of the virus into the cell and modification has been known for a long time that the CD4 located on the surface of T4 is contact with HIV surface protein, but this association was not enough to invade the cell and start life cycle for a long period of occupancy this acceptant ready to entry process for scientists around the world that was discovered recently by a research team from the National Institute of sensitivity and infectious diseases in the "Bethesda" state of Maryland. Named acceptant new (FUSIN) that this acceptant is a vehicle similar play the same role in different cells for different viral strains. There is no doubt that this evolutionary surge will continue, AIDS virus is still with us even more dangerous alleviation There is still room for creative contributions and creative, which is needed more than ever to join a global scientific effort to rid humanity of the plague of the twentieth century.

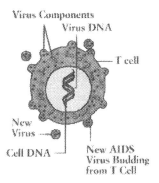

Virus Components
Virus DNA
T cell
New
Virus
Cell DNA
New AIDS
Virus Budding
from T Cell

AIDS infections are known as "opportunistic" because they are produced by commonplace organisms that do not trouble people whose immune systems are healthy, but which take advantage of the "opportunity" provided by an immune defense in disarray. The most common infection is an unusual and life-threatening form of pneumonia caused by a one-celled organism (a) called Pneumocystis carinii. AIDS patients are also **Protozoa** susceptible to unusual lymphomas and Kaposi's sarcoma, a rare cancer that results from the abnormal proliferation of endothelial cells in the blood vessels

Diagnosis of Viral Diseases

Diagnosis of viral diseases :-reliable diagnosis some viral diseases like influenza, measles and parotid gland on the patient's clinical symptoms, which show a clear, but some other diseases such as inflammation hepatitis and AIDS, the AIDS laboratory diagnosis, diagnosis is a necessity in this situation is by isolating the virus and identify it is a difficult issue requiring specialized labs a high level of processing and possibilities laboratory and trained human being or through diagnosis to confirm the existence of antibodies formed in the patient's blood to attack the virus and attempt to rid the body of knowledge and quantity analysis or radio-immunoassay kit. Because of the difficulty of growing viruses in cell cultures living lab or diagnosed by conventional means scientists have tended to use genetic engineering methods to detect viruses in the samples directly without turning to follow through segregation rules in the viral DNA known as a test enzyme polymerization reactions (PCR), the serial is important This test reveals that the least amount of the virus in the sample and thus the diagnosis of infection can occur at the beginning and is an important step in the early diagnosis of viral infection before the appearance of symptoms. For example, the crossing in the case of infection with hepatitis C distinct anti-virus composed after infection and continue during directly for a very long time even after recovery, in addition to that of the PCR test can determine the type of virus strain. The example reflects the importance of this is that it so far has been the discovery of five strains of HIV hepatitis C are not responding to treatment by interferon usual, thanks to identify race before treatment begins to be very costly addition to the side effects that no longer on the patient recovery. It is thus clear that the PCR test shows the picture before attending physician, which helped select the ideal method of treatment...

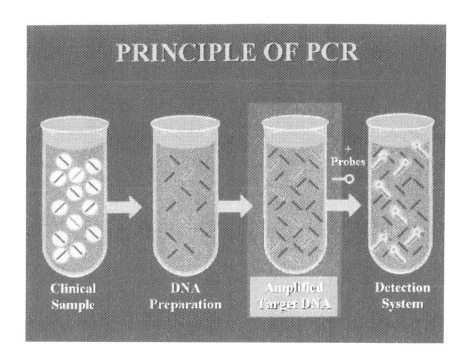

PRINCIPLE OF PCR

| Clinical Sample | DNA Preparation | Amplified Target DNA | Detection System |

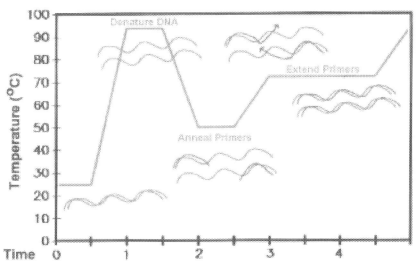

The Polymerase Chain Reaction (PCR)

Stem Cells

Stem cells :- embryonic stem cells and controversial cells multifaceted seem to be able to do anything has been expanded role in the prevention of cancer, the vaccine made of the two cells I prevention of rats from lung cancer in circumstances believed to simulate the impact of smoking. Fears that the safety of the injected human stem cell means it is unlikely to approve regulatory agencies to conduct tests on the vaccine on humans according to Dr. (Eaton) at the University of Louisville Kentucky state America. Despite this he believed that the vaccine deserves to be tested in people who have a high risk of cancer, such as smokers voracious or have certain genetic variations. Other researchers more careful, Vaccines against cancer, especially those made from cells known that the greatest impact on mice of Rights as saying "Jeffrey Webber," the wizard vaccine University of California at Los Angeles that the idea is interesting, but it seems that implementation was impossible. "But consistent, "Weber and Eaton," that the discovery may lead to new ways for prevent or treat cancer. The analogy between fetal and embryonic cells Torso brain tumors and insinuated that the idea of "Eaton," permanently, tumors grow both in the form of a ball and absorbing food from the host body, both proteins produced some strange commonplace. He says: these proteins made common Eaton believes that the protein stimulates the reaction of Immune Cells Stem embryonic brain and is also attacking tumors. The Eaton and his colleagues injected mice brain cells Torso then give booster after ten days, the researchers then planted Pulmonary cancer cells under the skin of animals, and after vaccination of mice showed that stem cell injury mice 20 out of 25 mice were tumor while all mice that had not been previously vaccinated. The most effective is the jumble of Stem cells and genetic engineering to make the molecule stimulates the immune system; none of these have been previously vaccinated mice tumor cells after transplant Cancer. this treatment also assessed mice 8 out of 9 mice from lung cancer caused by the chemical, which is believed to be similar to the impact of smoking. Although the mice did not suffer from any diseases result injected vaccine but "Eaton" recognizes that the injection of stem cells in human beings living raises topics such as safety if the vaccine makes the body attacking its stem cells. A team, "Eaton" Now molecules in the embryonic stem cells that would be granted the vaccine strength to kill tumor cells is likely to lead to a more effective vaccine against cancer and have a special vehicles. The best artistic dreams technical macroscopic NANOTECHNOLOGY'S is the presence of devices minutes searched body search of any strange objects invaded the body has a group of researchers in Israel device consisting of a molecule consisting of one molecule largely similar to those organs. They have built a "DNA machine that detects the virus through reading a genetic factor and then produces an alarm signal, in the form of a visible glow. But this system resembles very far from robot-dimensional macroscopic capable of killing the HIV virus-zapping "nanobot" at least because it needs to employ a range of other chemical elements were not the objective of making molecular robot innovation, but a new way of tracking the impact of viruses in a sample of blood for example. Say "Itamar willner" and his university Hebrew Jerusalem that the DNA device can reveal the virus during the hour and a half while other existing roads requires several complicated chemical steps for the detection of viruses or bacteria through DNA . say "Chengde Mao" competent in the field of IT miniatures macroscopic DNA University "purdue" state of Indiana, United States of America, "This how very sensitive". willner and his colleagues exploited the ability DNA test to work as a database of genetic and similar Enzyme catalyst to accelerate chemical reactions. that machine is a series of mono-molecular DNA contains three segments : the first is knowing sector A viruses found through DNA and the DNA sector C contains instructions for the manufacture of catalytic particles through DNA or DNA enzyme DNA either the third sector where B enrolled Enzyme and release the enzyme DNA from the rest of the molecule. this is how the system is a molecule of DNA test called Hairpin because its two ends close together to form a related through DNA of the bacterium in one of the parties and the sector A machine the other party, which stimulates the enzymes in the solution for building enzyme DNA encoded in the sector C and then cut to small pieces. The enzyme is known as (hemin) after activating enzyme DNA test that is transforming another molecule called (luminal) and makes a light.

Stem Cells

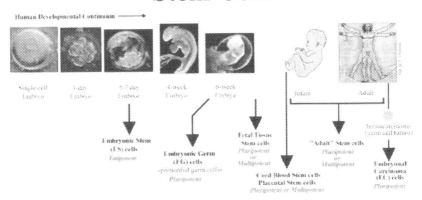

Human Developmental Continuum ──────▶

Single-cell Embryo | 3-day Embryo | 5-7 day Embryo | 4-week Embryo | 8-week Embryo | Infant | Adult

Embryonic Stem (ES) cells
Totipotent

Embryonic Germ (EG) cells
(primordial germ cells)
Pluripotent

Fetal Tissue Stem cells
Pluripotent or Multipotent

Cord Blood Stem cells Placental Stem cells
Pluripotent or Multipotent

"Adult" Stem cells
Pluripotent or Multipotent

Teratocarcinoma (germ cell tumor)

Embryonal Carcinoma (EC) cells
Pluripotent

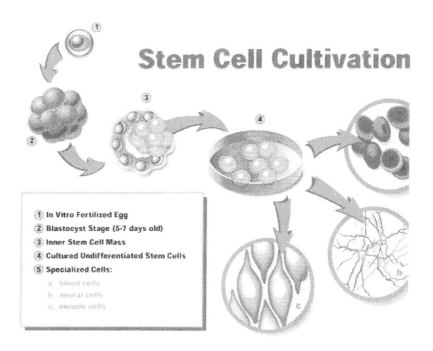

Stem Cell Cultivation

1. In Vitro Fertilized Egg
2. Blastocyst Stage (5-7 days old)
3. Inner Stem Cell Mass
4. Cultured Undifferentiated Stem Cells
5. Specialized Cells:
   a. blood cells
   b. neural cells
   c. muscle cells

Stem cell cultivation

1) In vitro fertilized egg - made in an artificial environment outside of a living organism.

2) Blastocyst stage - 5 to 7 days after egg is fertilized, cells are beginning to multiply.

3) Inner stem cell mass - removal of stem cells.

4) Cultured undifferentiated stem cells - stage when cells can be directed to what they will become.

5) Specialized cells - what the cells become.
a) blood cells
b) neural cells
c) muscle cells

Conclusion

Conclusion :—The great achievements in the field of biotechnological already served to deepen our understanding of the factors influencing the march of development and operations, especially those that have a significant impact in the evolution of the human race, people now know that some forms of advanced technology in the field of medicine and biological sciences were already available and could be used already and can be exploited in gene control as a lot of machines and technology complex, which brings us to the future, which allows us more room for governing gene widely after this, let alone the means available to us now that can be developed largely If books for humans to open new areas wider Bioethics It is the secret of development it can then increase the speed of evolutionary process or to modify the way in which it wishes. The scientists have consistently stressed that the progress of mankind depends on the progress of science free hand search, but they quickly for the laboratories and devised us artificial distinction between science and the results, after what appeared visible risk imposed on the path of science and misdeeds of applications that resulted in either the biggest proof of the weakness of feature neutrality in contemporary science, it is the pressure that surround it in the present day, the path taken by the flag meant originally that option was available to move in this way without this, but make science take the road means that there is a specific point of what it wanted to walk in the knowledge that point without the other. It is not in the course of science inevitable or that it is impossible to put an end to it, because it is quite possible through the monitoring of the budget for scientific research admiration, but the issue here that the financial budget of fun for science can not be free from ideological considerations example, or specific values or preferences self wants to learn that much compared to the money that is spent. Whatever it is the factor of funding and spending on scientific research is only one side of the issue-the issue of neutrality in science-an external factor is the pressure on the face of science and nature from abroad, but there is another factor is the internal responsibility of scientists and researchers about future developments in the fields of science The impact on human progress, or delay..

References

1-Ball; Philip: "A designed DNA molecule lights up when it   spots a pathogen"(DNA machine sounds the virus alert), published online :10 November 2006 . news@nature.com

2-Ainsworth; Claire: "Experimental cystic-fibrosis treatment could be used in many diseases"(drug makes cells ignore mutation). Published online, 9 November 2006; news@nature.com

3-Schubert; charlotte: "cancer vaccine harnesses similarities between embryos and tumors (stem cells fend off lung cancer), published online: 10 November 2006; news@nature.com

4-Content.answer.com/topic/gene-therapy.

5-Monogenic forms of diabetics: neonatal diabetes mellitus and maturity-onset diabetes of young diabetes –niddk. nih .gov /dm/pub/ mody/

6-www.benbest.com/lifeext/DNA repairs Genes. Jpg.

7- erl.pathology.iupui.edu/C603/Gene 195. HTM.

8-www.nature.com /nm/web specials /Xenon /review. Html.

9-www.seafriends.org.nz/issues/cons/conserve.htm.

10-www.medscape.com/view article /416519-25. (Lieberman/slide08. gif).

11- Swahel, Dr. Wagdi Abdel-Fattah. (Gene bank). Science magazine (Academy of Scientific Research and Technology-Egypt) (226). In July 1995, pages 6,7,11.

12- Fishawi, Dr. Fawzi Abdul Qadir. (Genes dealing with the environment). Science magazine (Academy of Scientific Research and Technology-Egypt) (229). In October 1995, pages 42-45.

13- Faraj, Dr. Najib Nashaat. (Genetic engineering medicine tomorrow). Science magazine (Academy of Scientific Research and Technology-Egypt) (247). In April 1997, pages 46,47.

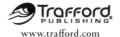

www.trafford.com

North America & international
toll-free: 1 888 232 4444 (USA & Canada)
phone: 250 383 6864 ♦ 812 355 4082

Printed in the United States
By Bookmasters